I0429909

Essentials Of Essential Oils

Essentials of Essential Oils

How to Use Essential Oils for Beginners

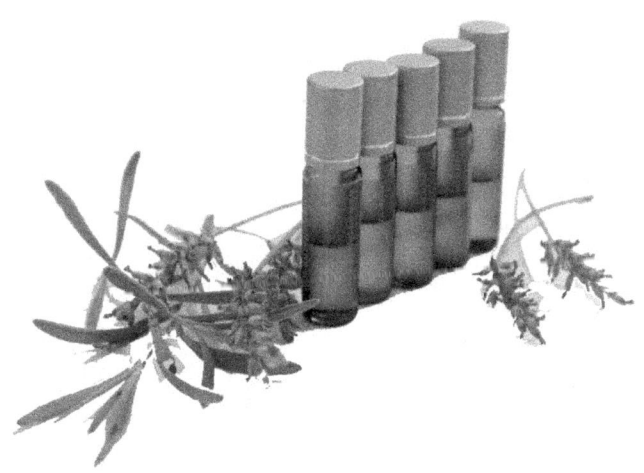

Rachel Ramey

DISCLAIMER: I am not a medical professional, and none of the statements in this book have been evaluated by the FDA. The information in this book is presented for educational purposes only, and nothing here should be construed as diagnosing, treating, or preventing any illness or condition. As always, please exercise your own judgment and common sense.

© 2014 Rachel B. Ramey
All rights reserved.
No part of this publication may be reproduced in any form or by any means without the prior written permission of the author, except for brief quotations for the purpose of reviews.

CONTENTS

INTRODUCTION

Essential oils are becoming better- and better-known as an option for home health care. But there is still an air of mystery about them, as so few people seem to know what to do with them. People wonder how to use them safely. They wonder which oils they need. They wonder whose information to believe.

This confusion is due, in large part, to our having lost the tradition somewhere along the way. We're now having to re-learn what used to be passed down informally. In this booklet, I hope to provide some foundational information about essential oils and their use that will help you to make sense of the other information you read.

This is by no means an exhaustive volume! There is not a lot of information here about individual oils or specific health concerns. Rather, this is the information that will provide a framework for all those *other* books that tell you what to use when. Think of this as the "big picture" that will enable you to put the details into their proper context.

BEGINNING AT THE BEGINNING: WHAT IS AN ESSENTIAL OIL?

Contrary to what the name implies, an essential oil is not really an "oil." It isn't greasy. It won't leave oil stains. In layman's terms, an essential oil is the non-water-soluble elements of the plant matter when distilled (usually by the use of steam) into concentrated form.

As nice as the idea is, you can't make your own essential oil at home. A home distillery is not inexpensive, and it takes a *lot* of plant matter to make a little bit of oil. (On the order of 100's of pounds of plant for 1 pound of oil.)

When you find ebooks or websites that claim to teach you to make your own essential oil, what they're really showing is *infused* oils. These can be useful for some purposes, but they are not interchangeable with essential oils.

Essential oils have several traits that contribute to their effectiveness. From an energetic perspective, they have very high frequencies, which can (somehow; I don't understand it!) help bring the body into a better balance when it's unwell. (Energy medicine is still poorly understood, but more and more, the research is showing that tradition lines up with science.)

Many of the reasons for essential oils' effectiveness are not so "ethereal," though. For one thing, an essential oil is very (very!) highly concentrated. For another, the molecular structure is so tiny that it can pass certain "barriers" within the body that other substances have difficulty crossing – things like cell walls and the blood-brain barrier. This allows the beneficial qualities of the essential oil's constituents (things with fancy chemical names like terpenes, monoterpenes, and phenols) to get to the places in the body where they can do their work.

WHY ESSENTIAL OILS AS OPPOSED TO HERBS?

Why use essential oil? Why not just use herbs? There are a few reasons.

First, there is the concentrated nature of the oils. Not only does this make them quite potent, it makes them *space-saving*. Three dozen essential oils could easily be stored in a shoebox. Try storing three dozen herbs in that same space! You wouldn't have much to work with.

Second, they're easily portable and simple to use. You don't have to make decoctions or poultices or strain anything or throw piles of soaked, "used-up" herbs into the compost heap.

There's more to it than that, though. Most people who use herbs concentrate on decoctions – essentially herbal "teas." But remember I said earlier that essential oils are the *non*-water-soluble components of the plant? Well, a decoction will draw out the *water-soluble* elements. If you're using an herb or you're using the essential oil from the same plant, you're getting two entirely different things, in terms of the effective constituents. I don't believe one is good and one is bad. Both can be beneficial; they're just different.

THREE SCHOOLS OF THOUGHT

When you begin to study essential oils, you'll quickly find that much of the information is contradictory. That can be exceptionally frustrating for someone just starting out, who simply wants a straight answer! The vast majority of the disagreement arises from the fact that there are three separate "schools" of aromatherapy, each with a different philosophy. (These "schools" are schools of thought, not specific institutions.) Material written by a proponent of one philosophy will tend to conflict with material written by a proponent of a different school of thought. Understanding which one your reading material reflects will help prevent confusion.

The **German** school of aromatherapy relies primarily on *inhalation* of the essential oils. Perhaps because it's so limited in scope, we don't often hear about/from this one.

The **French** school of aromatherapy emphasizes the internal use of oils & the "neat" application of oils. (It's okay if you don't really know what that means! I will explain in a later chapter.) It also makes use of inhalation, massage with diluted essential oils, and suppositories.

These two schools arose primarily for *therapeutic* purposes, and therefore find their emphases in therapeutic uses. The French school, as you may have gathered, places little limitation on how the oils may be used, making use of pretty much any delivery option available.

The **British** school of aromatherapy emphasizes the use of only diluted oils – usually at a dilution rate of 2-5%. It specifically discourages the use of essential oils "neat" or internally, and generally uses only single oils (not blends).

This school arose for purposes that were primarily connected with massage and emotional well-being or relaxation, making use of fragrance- or food-grade oils (not therapeutic-grade). The warnings typically given by this school make perfect sense in light of the *quality* of oils in use within it. (You might think that "food-grade" would be a good thing, but that designation may indicate that the oil has been altered to fit within certain parameters that are easier to regulate.)

METHODS OF APPLICATION/USE

As the last chapter indicated, essential oils can be used several different ways. You can sniff them straight out of the bottle (like smelling salts). You can rub them onto the skin, either diluted (in another, *real* oil) or, in many cases, "neat" (undiluted). You can diffuse them into the air. And in some cases, you can ingest them.

But you have to make sure you're safe about it! Different oils have different characteristics, and not every one is safe for use in every manner. (As far as I know, practically every essential oil that's safe for human application is safe to diffuse, so if you're in doubt, that's your best bet.)

Some people say you should never use them neat and/or that you should never ingest them. You'll have to do your own research of course, and decide what you're personally comfortable with, but now you know that these warnings are largely dependent on which school the speaker/writer is from – and the quality of your oils.

If you aren't sure of the purity of your oils, I would definitely avoid ingesting them or using them neat. Be aware, though, that most essential oil companies in the United States will *officially* tell you they don't recommend ingesting their oils. I'm pretty sure that's for legal reasons more than health reasons. Some of them very well may ingest the oils themselves.

If you do choose to ingest essential oils or use them neat, be sure you know which ones are *un*safe to ingest (or should not be used neat). And keep in mind how highly concentrated they are. We're talking *drops*, not teaspoons!

Some oils are "hot" and should always be diluted. Some aren't safe for consumption (although they're just fine externally). And a few oils will make the skin particularly photosensitive and you'll need to be careful of sun (or other UV) exposure for a little while after use. But with some common sense and some basic research, the use of essential oils can be very safe!

- **Topical Application of Essential Oils, Neat**

"Neat" is the term for an essential oil used "straight," undiluted. It's the simplest and most straightforward method of use, so we'll start here. To apply an essential oil neat, you would simply take a drop or two of the oil and rub it into the skin.

Unless you're applying it for a particular localized issue (like a cut or a burn), the most common places to apply the oil are the chest or the soles of the feet. You can vary this, though, based on common sense or intuition. For a headache, apply the oil to the temples. Oils are also sometimes applied to earlobes, pulse points, or along the spine. (The chest and feet are usually pretty accessible, though, even if you're applying them to yourself.)

Precautions: Some oils are "hot" and should never be applied neat, but always diluted. Notable common oils that are hot oils are peppermint, oregano, cinnamon, basil, cedarwood, clove, and possibly rosemary. (As a general rule of thumb, if the plant it's derived from is a "spicy" food, it will be a hot oil. Although, as you can see, there are others.) If a blend includes a hot oil, it will probably be a hot blend.

(Your personal experience may vary. I've known a few people who have used some of these hot oils neat, so use your discretion, but be advised! If you apply an oil neat – or with minimal dilution – and it *does* become too hot, you can alleviate the discomfort by rubbing carrier oil onto the skin in the same location.)

Some oils are photosensitive. What we mean by that, really, is that they *cause* photosensitivity. When these oils are applied topically (either neat or diluted), they increase the skin's sensitivity to the sun (or other UV light) for several hours to as much as a day (depending on the person) following application. Citrus oils are photosensitive. Citrus oils include bergamot (strongly photosensitive), as well as the others you'd probably recognize as citrus, like lemon and mandarin.

- **Topical Application of Essential Oils, Diluted**

If you're dealing with a hot oil or a sensitive individual, or if you're just not comfortable using oils neat, you can dilute them. Oils are not water-soluble, remember, so we don't dilute them in water. We dilute them in oil. The oils we use for dilution are referred to as "carrier oils," because they "carry" the essential oils to their intended locations. We'll talk more about carrier oils in a later chapter.

Precautions: Note the warning above regarding photosensitivity.

- **Diffusion of Essential Oils**

To diffuse something means, in essence, to "spread it out" throughout a space. So when we talk about diffusing an essential oil, we are talking about taking it from a small space - wherever your few drops of essential oil are – and distributing it throughout the surrounding air.

There are a handful of different types of diffusion (different methods that accomplish the "spreading out"), but some are better than others. Heat diffusion, for instance, will *work*, but it isn't recommended because the heat alters the chemical composition of the oil, so what you end up with in your air may not be quite the same thing you put in your diffuser.

(This is probably okay if you're just using small amounts for the sake of a pleasant scent, but for therapeutic purposes it will not be very effective. And with less-mainstream oils, it may occasionally not be as safe.)

Cold air nebulizers blow the oil into a nebulizer for dispersion. These are okay, but may not effectively diffuse thicker, heavier oils.

The best option is an ultrasonic diffuser. This uses frequency waves to vibrate the essential oils, which float on the surface of a small quantity of water in a chamber, and the vibrations break up the oil so it can be dispersed. The only downside to this type of diffuser is that because of the water it also releases moisture. Normally this isn't a problem, but if you're trying to deal with mold or a similar issue, you might prefer a cold air nebulizer.

- **Inhalation of Essential Oils**

Diffusion technically is a form of inhalation, since you're diffusing the oils into the air you then *breathe*. But in an even simpler manner, you can use the oils by simply *sniffing* them.

We also benefit from inhalation of essential oils whenever they're used for scenting products like bath salts, candles, or lip balm. (Note that some of these also result in absorption through the skin, which is topical. And lip balm may end up in the mouth, so pay attention to ingestibility of oils used for lip balms.)

Precautions: If it's a hot oil, don't get too close!

- **Massage with Essential Oils**

A variation on topical application is to add essential oils to your lotions or oils for massage.

Precautions: The same precautions used for topical application. Be aware of proper dilutions if massaging babies or small children, and any pregnancy-related precautions for pregnancy massage.

- **Ingestion of Essential Oils**

The safety of ingesting essential oils is more hotly debated than perhaps any other issue regarding these oils. For most purposes, I don't personally see any *need* to take essential oils internally, so my first recommendation would be to use another method if the other method will effectively accomplish your goal.

If you do choose to use oils internally, be sure you have a very pure, unadulterated, unaltered, high-quality oil and that it's a variety that's safe for ingestion. (If it's from a part of a plant that's typically food, it's probably okay. But that's a general rule; be sure to verify any oil you're consuming!)

Essential oils are not water-soluble, but you can put a drop or two in about half of a cup of water, shake it up, and drink it *immediately* if you need to take it internally. (Peppermint is sometimes used this way for an upset stomach.)

They can be taken by placing a drop or two in a capsule and taking it with water. (This would need to be used right away, as well, because the oil will start to dissolve your capsule if you leave it to sit.)

They can be added to honey or honey + water as a means of taking them internally.

Some can also be used to flavor foods. (Pay attention to quantity. Remember that these are *very* concentrated, so check any recipe before use to make sure it doesn't result in an unreasonably high "dosage.")

Precautions: *Never* consume essential oils undiluted. Use a strong dose of common sense when determining quantities. (You should definitely not be consuming more than a couple of drops of essential oil at any given time.) And check to be certain ingestion of a given variety of oil is not contraindicated first!

- **Essential Oil Suppositories**

Suppositories are probably the least common method of essential oil use here in the United States (or close to it). And I wouldn't recommend that you *start* here! But this is a not-uncommon method of application in the French school of aromatherapy.

Suppositories bypass the liver and, oddly enough, oils utilized in this way are more efficiently delivered to the *lungs* than ingested oils.

(Who would have thought? It has to do with the circulatory pathways, though, of things absorbed abdominally.)

The "trick" to a suppository is using a carrier that will melt to liquid in order to incorporate the essential oil, solidify to allow for insertion, and then melt again to release the oils. Dr. Kurt Schnaubelt suggests a 2/3 cocoa butter, 1/3 "liquid oil" blend, and an approximate 10% dilution of essential oils (for adults; use less for children).

When everything is melted together, let it partially harden, roll up in aluminum foil, and freeze to harden fully.

Precautions: All of the relevant precautions from other portions of this chapter, applied using common sense!

Other Safety Concerns (Including Essential Oil Use for Babies and Pregnant Women)

There is some debate over certain safety issues – either of essential oils in general, or specifically regarding use by pregnant or nursing women or application to babies. Some sources actually recommend oils that others specify to avoid!

There are several reasons for this:

- Some recommendations are based on studies of adulterated/altered oils or essential oils' lab-derived counterparts. These may or may not be valid when applied to true, pure essential oils.
- Some recommendations come from extrapolation based on herbal actions. That is, if an herb is considered to have a certain action, the essential oil from the same plant is assumed to have the same action. This may or may not be accurate, because the composition of the herb and the essential oil are different (as mentioned in chapter 1).
- Some recommendations vary because of the differing schools of thought. Proponents of the British school often

recommend against things proponents of the French school *recommend*.

- Some are simply being overly cautious, acting on the adage that it's better to be safe than sorry. (Not necessarily a bad thing!)
- Finally, there are a few legitimate concerns to be aware of.

Keep this context in mind, and you can make your own wise judgment calls.

Babies and small children have more sensitive skin, and (obviously!) tinier bodies. This means that a little goes a long way (even more so than with adults), and that oils that don't cause irritation on adult skin may well irritate theirs. Common sense dictates, then, that when working with children we use less and dilute more. Some of the hottest oils we might opt not to use at all with young children.

Pregnant women also have more sensitive – and more permeable-than-usual – skin. Many essential oils can cross the placental barrier just as they do other barriers within the body. So caution is needed here, too. Again, increased dilution is probably wise. And use your own best judgment when it comes to *which* oils to use.

Many warnings about particular oils in pregnancy are probably exaggerated. Evidence suggests that oils would have to be *very* heavily applied or taken in unreasonable quantities by mouth to cause a real issue with miscarriage or toxicity for the baby. Many recommendations are probably based more on *lack* of proof that a given oil is safe, rather than the *existence* of evidence that it's unsafe. But use your judgment and be wise.

Personally, when it comes to herbs or essential oils, I will pay a lot of attention to how *long* a given oil or herb has been in use. If the Chinese have been using something for 3,000 years without ill effect, I might not care that we don't have a clinical study for it. If, on the other hand, the herb/oil is not well-known, I find it wiser to pass (particularly in terms of safety during pregnancy). As Chrissie

Wildwood says in *The Encyclopedia of Aromatherapy,* "Never use an essential oil about which you can find little or no information."

According to Dr. Kurt Schnaubelt, essential oils high in potentially hazardous ketones include sage, mugwort, thuja, (some varieties of) *Hyssop officinalis*, and *Lavendula stoechas* (not to be confused with *Lavendula angustifolia*). These legitimately present a concern, and are probably best avoided by laypeople entirely. (Several are available in specific varieties which circumvent the problematic constituents, but this is not something you'll want to approach with insufficient knowledge.)

Dr. Schnaubelt also suggests that citrus, needle-based (like pine), and tea tree oils may be prone to peroxidation, in which case they *might* present an increased likelihood of irritating the skin (this appears to be an issue – or non-issue – that varies from individual to individual, and it should be less of a likelihood the fresher your oil); cinnamon and clove oils may be more likely than average to cause sensitization if used topically, especially at higher dilutions; and thyme, oregano, or savory may be more likely than many other oils to be irritants to certain individuals. None of the issues in this paragraph is a *serious* concern, so it should be sufficient to be aware so *if* something comes up, you have a better idea what you're dealing with.

As a final safety precaution, don't get essential oils in your eyes. If you do, you'll want to flush them out.

HOW TO CHOOSE QUALITY ESSENTIAL OILS

Of particular importance when using essential oils therapeutically –
especially if they're to be used neat or (even more especially)
internally – is ensuring that your oils are of high quality. Some
companies will tell you that they are the *only* sellers of truly pure,
good quality oils. I don't believe this is true. However, I do believe
you have to be careful about your source(s).

Essential oils are expensive to produce, so there's a good deal of
financial incentive to adulterate them. And there are many ways to
do so. This means that buying good oils can, unfortunately, be a little
tricky.

We want oils that are distilled properly, not subjected to too much
heat, not "washed" with chemicals, not "cut" with anything, and with
nothing added. That's fairly *simple*, but there are a number of stages
during the process where this can be derailed.

What makes it particularly difficult is that the average home user
doesn't really have any way to be *certain* that what his supplier is
telling him is the truth. Even mass spectrometry testing (which most
of us can't do at home!) has limited use, because it can only tell us
which compounds are present – and there are only certain ones they
actually check for. (Lots of trace elements are just that – trace. Like
in good quality salt, they matter. But they're not necessarily easy to
nail down.)

All of this means that the key to getting a good oil is to choose a
reputable supplier. Ideally, a company will tell you, *for each oil*, what
its botanical name is, where it came from (country of origin, for
instance), by what method it was distilled, and what part(s) of the
plant was/were used. They might not all publish this directly on their
websites, but they should all be able to tell you if/when you ask.

Although we can't, as individual consumers, actually *test* the oils at home to see if they meet the sellers' claims (unfortunately!), there are some things we can do at home that can give us *some* idea and that will indicate *clearly* bad oils. And there are things we can know to look for (and ask about) that can be a very good start.

Labeling Claims

The first difficulty is that certain claims you'll often see on a label or description either don't mean anything (from a standardized/legal standpoint), or don't necessarily mean what you would expect them to. Some of you may be familiar with this concept from dealing with food labels. "Wheat bread" is a relatively meaningless term when shopping for bread. The savvy consumer knows to look for "100% wheat bread" if she wants what the average person refers to as "wheat bread."

A manufacturer's claim that an essential oil is "100% pure" is similar. This means only that *the portion of the contents which are essential oils* is unadulterated/-altered. The essential oil can still be "cut" with a large proportion of a carrier oil and bear this claim. (I think that as much as 90% of the bottle can actually be carrier oil, but don't quote me on that number. Suffice it to say, we're not talking 1-2%.)

"Therapeutic grade" is another virtually useless label. In theory, "therapeutic grade" would mean that the oil is of good quality, unaltered, unadulterated, uncontaminated, uncut, and safe for internal use. In actuality, it doesn't mean anything at all. It isn't a regulated term, so companies toss it around to make their oils sound good. But this "therapeutic grade" oil may or may not be what you'd hope to get.

"Natural" and "organic" don't mean what the average consumer expects them to mean, either. "Natural" can, for instance, mean "completely manufactured in a laboratory to mimic a truly natural compound." Yes, really. (This is true of "natural flavors" in your food, too, by the way.) And "organic" may just as well be *mineral*-based as *plant*-based.

So why bother with labels? What *is* meaningful? Well, there are some things you'll find on labels that you know you *don't* want. You *don't* want "aromatherapy grade." By definition, this means it's diluted in carrier oils. You don't want "USP grade," or "BP grade," which, by definition, mean the oils are laboratory-altered to meet specific, consistent standards.

What you *do* want is likely not on the label, and you may have to do a little digging to find it out. (These are the things you'll need to ask your supplier about, if the supplier doesn't specify.)

- **You want an oil that is essential oil *only*, with no carrier oil or anything else added to dilute it.** (You can dilute it for *use*, depending on your purpose, but you don't want to pay for "essential oil" that's already diluted.)
- **You want an oil that is distilled without chemicals and, as much as possible, without heat.** With a few rare exceptions, you want it to be either steam distilled (and from the *first* distillation), or CO2-distilled. (There are a few plants whose essential oils cannot be extracted by these more common means, but they are the exception, not the rule. Citrus oils are distilled from the citrus *peels*, and they are legitimately extracted by cold-pressing.)
- **You want an oil that is considered safe to take internally.** Although the recommendations vary, and although you may not *choose* to ever use them internally, a company's telling you their oils are *safe* for internal use should confirm a certain minimal degree of purity.

- **You want to buy from a company that is well aware of the path their oils take from grower to distiller to them.** There are any number of ways that an oil may be altered or adulterated along the way – even to the point of manipulating lab testing – and your supplier will have no way of knowing this if they aren't intimately familiar with *their* suppliers.
- **You need to be able to *trust* your supplier.** As noted earlier, we do not have the capability to fully test our oils at home to be sure we're not being lied to, so you will have to trust your supplier's honesty.

"Testing" Your Oils

There are a couple basic things you can test, that will help to turn up *obviously* altered oils. The first relates to the fact that essential oils aren't true oils. They shouldn't leave oil stains, so if you put a drop of your oil on a piece of paper and it leaves an oily spot after a couple of days, the oil has been diluted. (Do note that some essential oils are interesting *colors*. Don't confuse the color with an oily place. And note that it takes some time for the oils to completely evaporate – some more than others.)

Second, a good essential oil will have a multitude of molecular components. This means that it will also have different layers of *scent*. Smell the (uncapped) bottle with it near your nose (not *too* close, though, if it's a "hot" oil like peppermint!). Then move it about six inches lower and sniff again. Repeat.

Does the oil smell exactly the same every time? Or do you notice a subtle change as the distance increases? If it stays exactly the same, it could be that your oil has been "fiddled with" to maintain certain levels of particular components, but doesn't have the full natural bouquet. (Or it could just be that you don't have a very discerning sense of smell. Ask a family member to repeat the test.)

Third, do the oils work? Ultimately, *this* is the big test. If they don't do what they're supposed to do, maybe your oils aren't of a very good quality.

(Note that the first two "tests" are only general guidelines. They'll give you a better idea if you're looking at a fairly wide selection of one company's oils as compared to another, rather than an individual oil, because each variety of essential oil has its own quirks.)

The most important thing is to find a supplier that seems to be trustworthy (and to know what they're doing).

CARRIER OILS

When diluting essential oils for use, we typically use carrier oils – that is, true oils. A larger quantity of true oil is used to "carry" a smaller quantity of essential oil to the place you want it.

There are many options, and all the unfamiliar names of not-so-common oils can get overwhelming, but it really doesn't have to be complicated! Pretty much any oil you would eat/rub on your skin can be used as a carrier oil. If you're just getting started, that's enough.

A few examples of oils that can be used as carriers include:

- Coconut oil
- Fractionated coconut oil (This is a popular oil to use as a carrier. Certain parts of the oil have been removed so the oil stays liquid, unlike "regular" coconut oil, which solidifies at just below body temperature. This also has an indefinite shelf life; it doesn't readily oxidize/go rancid. "MCT" oil is just another name for this, although it appears that "MCT" is often used for food-grade oil, while "fractionated coconut oil" is often used for oil that isn't approved for consumption.)
- Olive oil (This might smell/look a little weird for topical use, but it works just fine, so if you have it in your kitchen, go for it!)
- Sweet almond oil*
- Walnut oil*
- Grapeseed oil
- Jojoba oil (Pronounced ho-HO-buh, this oil closely mimics the natural human skin/hair oils, so it's excellent when you want something non-greasy-feeling for skin or hair applications. It also has mildly preservative properties, so it can be good to add to blends of other oils that you want to "keep" a little better.)

- Hazelnut oil*
- Avocado oil

*Be aware of allergies when using tree nut oils!

Liquid oils like those above can be combined with "butters" and such when you need a thicker end product. (For example, shea butter, cocoa butter, or beeswax) These butters and waxes tend to be too thick on their own, though.

(Remember to watch for allergies here, too. Many "butters" are tree-nut based, and they're often not very familiar, so you might need to do some checking if you are dealing with an allergic person.)

In a pinch, all kinds of things can be used as carriers. Anything you would apply to your skin will work. Maybe you don't have any oil handy, but you have some lotion. Body washes and bubble baths can "carry" essential oils into a bath.

Other non-oil carriers can be used, as well, depending on the intended application.

- **Aloe** can be applied to the skin, or used in combination with other ingredients for hair or body products.
- **Glycerin** can be used to apply something to the skin (although it probably wouldn't be my first choice on its own, as it's mildly sticky) or in combination with other ingredients in hair or body products. It's water- and alcohol-soluble, and can help your essential oils to distribute through water if you want them for a spritz or something.
- **Water** is not a good carrier for general purposes because the essential oils won't mix with it, but it can be used under certain circumstances. If you're taking a couple drops internally, water can serve as a carrier if you shake it up and drink immediately. Or it can sometimes be mixed in with other ingredients to thin a concoction.

- **Witch hazel** is not for internal consumption, but may be used in hair or body products.
- **Vodka or other alcohol** is a similar option.
- **Honey** is sometimes a beneficial addition to hair or body products. It's also safe for internal consumption (after toddlerhood) and can help distribute essential oils through water more effectively.
- "Dry ingredients" like **Epsom salts, sea salt, baking soda, Bentonite clay, etc.** can also be used. For something like this – if you're not mixing them with liquids – you will typically add a few drops of essential oil to a larger quantity of the dry ingredient, shake well to distribute, and allow to sit for a while (covered), shaking again periodically so you can be sure the oils are evenly distributed throughout the product. Note that these are for *external* applications.

The following dilution chart should be helpful if you're just getting started. The recommended percentages are merely guidelines. As you get more familiar, you may be comfortable with moving outside of the recommended ranges. But they provide a safe starting point.

(If you want a printable version of the chart, see the back of this book.)

Essential Oil Dilution Guide

Carrier Oil Qty.	.1%	.25%	.5%	1%	1.5%	2%	2.5%	3%	5%
1 tsp.*	n/a	n/a	n/a	1	*1.5*	2	*2.5*	3	5
2 tsp.	n/a	n/a	1	2	3	4	5	6	10
3 tsp. (1 Tbsp.)	n/a	n/a	*1.5*	3	*4.5*	6	*7.5*	9	15
4 tsp.	n/a	1	2	4	6	8	10	12	20
5 tsp.	n/a	*1.25*	*2.5*	5	*7.5*	10	*12.5*	15	25
6 tsp. (2 Tbsp.)	n/a	*1.5*	3	6	9	12	15	18	30
7 tsp.	n/a	*1.75*	*3.5*	7	*10.5*	14	*17.5*	21	35
8 tsp.	n/a	2	4	8	12	16	20	24	40
9 tsp. (3 Tbsp.)	n/a	*2.25*	*4.5*	9	*13.5*	18	*22.5*	27	45
10 tsp.	1	*2.5*	5	10	15	20	25	30	50

Key: The left column is the carrier oil quantity. The top row is the dilution.
The intersecting boxes show the number of drops of essential oil needed for that dilution in that quantity of carrier oil.
Pink italicized numbers are quantities which include partial drops.
n/a indicates less than 1 drop.

Helpful Equivalents
20 drops = 1 ml
5 ml = 1 tsp.
3 tsp. = 1 Tbsp.
2 Tbsp. = 1 fl oz.

*If you have trouble remembering the numbers, just remember this!
At 1 teaspoon of carrier oil, 1 drop of essential oil = 1%
(100 drops = 1 tsp.)

Suggested Dilutions:

NB-3 mos.: .1 - .2%   6-15 yrs.: 1.5 – 3%
3-24 mos.: .25 - .5%   15+:   2.5 – 5%
2-6 yrs.:   1 - 2%

Keep in mind these are all *guidelines*. Use your own best judgment.

HOW TO STORE ESSENTIAL OILS

Properly-stored essential oils will last a long time. Citrus oils can lose their potency after about a year or so, but other oils last much longer. There are differing opinions on just how long. Some say they are good indefinitely. Others say they decrease in potency over time and/or eventually begin to oxidize and become rancid. It does seem probable that the efficacy of an oil will gradually decline over time. However, most sources agree that a non-citrus oil should be good and effective for *at least* 5-10 years if properly stored.

What does properly-stored mean? In short, it means protected from light, air, and heat. In practical terms, that means store your oils tightly capped, in dark jars, in a location that isn't too hot. (Blue or amber glass bottles are usually the preferred containers.)

Do not store your essential oils in plastic or they will eat/dissolve the plastic! (I know, that sounds kind of scary. It has to do with the *composition* of essential oils and the composition of plastic. It doesn't mean they're caustic or anything.)

Dropper bottles and roller bottles are both available. Roller bottles are especially good for prediluted oils (or oils you plan to use neat) because they make it very easy to apply without spillage.

The bottles are tiny, so it helps to gather them all together on a tray or in a small basket or bin. Ice cube trays are a good option, too. The individual compartments allow you to keep the jars from clanking together. Hexagonal ice trays make an excellent use of the space. However, any with large enough wells to accommodate your jars will work. There's a smaller hexagonal one that's a perfect size for the smaller roller vials. (The standard dropper bottles are too large to fit in it.) Drawer dividers are another option for corralling oil bottles.

Once you've accumulated a number of oils, you might want to invest in a special rack and/or case designed specifically for holding essential oils. Of course, it's totally up to you!

Once you have all of your oils on a tray or in a basket, the regular labels will be a little hard to see. It helps to get labels for the *lids*, so you can glance at the tops of all your bottles and see what everything is.

WHAT OILS TO START WITH

I don't want to get into a lot of specifics in this book, because there are dozens of books already out there that have plenty of specific details regarding which oils are beneficial for what purposes. I don't want to produce unnecessary "noise" in the information arena! But I do want to give you a starting point.

My personal recommendation is to start with three single oils and, if you can afford it, one blend. The three singles I recommend for a starter kit are:

- Peppermint
- Lavender
- Lemon

(If you can afford to add one blend, I'd add a "four thieves"-style blend. This is a highly disinfectant blend modeled after herbs used by four thieves during the Bubonic Plague to protect themselves against infection while they robbed bodies! It goes by different names depending on the company – the one I use is called "Shield" – and it's handy to have around as a "big guns" disinfectant.)

Why do I recommend these three oils, in particular? As essential oils go, they're inexpensive, so they're pretty accessible. They're somewhat "familiar," so they aren't intimidating for "newbies." They're all very safe, without any unusual warnings, so they're not too scary for starting out. (Peppermint should not be used undiluted, but apart from that, they can all be used with any application method.) And with just those three oils, you can tackle almost any basic first aid/home health/household need: headache, fevers, nausea, cough/congestion, cuts/scrapes, burns, pest deterring, cleaning/disinfecting...

Peppermint (*Mentha piperita*) is analgesic (meaning it's mildly pain-reducing), antibacterial, anti-inflammatory, antiseptic, and antiviral.

It's useful for congestion & respiratory concerns, cold sores, constipation, nausea & indigestion, fevers, flu, allergies, headache, and itching. It's beneficial in cleaning supplies, and rodents and ants typically don't like it.

Lavender (*Lavendula angustifolia*) is analgesic, antidepressant, antifungal, antihistamine, anti-inflammatory, antimicrobial, antiseptic, and sedative (that means calming/soothing, not "knock you out"!)

It's useful for acne, cuts & scrapes, blisters, sunburn, burns, itching, poison ivy, hives, chicken pox, impetigo, measles, mumps, allergy, thrush, ADD, stress, headaches, nausea & indigestion, teething, and repelling bugs. It is also frequently used in cleaning supplies.

Lemon (*Citrus limon*) is antidepressant, antiseptic, antifungal, antiviral, astringent, and invigorating/tonic.

It is useful for viruses, anxiety, fevers, autism, concentration, colds, sore throats, congestion & respiratory concerns, anemia/blood disorders, heartburn, ulcers, kidney stones, malaria, mumps, and stress. It is also beneficial for air purification, cleaning supplies (including disinfecting, polishing furniture, and "gunk" removal), and possibly even water purification.

As you can see, these three oils comprise quite a household tool chest!

A FEW PRACTICAL TIPS

Here are a few random practical tips and tidbits that didn't fit anywhere else.

If you're planning to use an oil diluted, it can be handy to dilute it *right in the bottle*. That will save you having to mix it up every time. (Be sure you'll use it within a reasonable period of time, though – say, 6 months or so – because the carrier oil can go rancid with time.)

Roller vial tops generally will pop off if you need them to. The ball doesn't come out - the whole plastic assembly does.

If you need a dilution for short-term use, baby food jars can be a handy container for mixing in. You can close them up so dust doesn't get in and keep them for two or three days. (You don't want to store your oil this way long-term, because the clear glass doesn't block out light, but for a few days it should be fine.)

Shot glasses are another mixing option, if you're using something right away.

Keep in mind that natural personal care products will go rancid, so if you're making these products yourself, they won't last indefinitely. It's a good thing to not have all the chemical preservatives in our products, but it does mean they have a shelf life, so be aware. (And if you're selling something, it's best to put an expiration date on it.) Items with a lot of moisture in them (like lotions) can also mold eventually.

Although essential oils don't go rancid – at least, not within any reasonable period of time – most *real* oils *do*. So don't expect to store your carrier oils indefinitely, either.

You can use clay to make pendants and let it dry/harden. Then put a drop of essential oil on the pendant and let the clay absorb it. This is a handy way to benefit from inhalation of an oil.

FOR FURTHER READING

Are you interested in learning more? Check out these titles:

- **anything by Robert B. Tisserand**
- *The Encyclopedia of Aromatherapy*, by Chrissie Wildwood
- *The Healing Intelligence of Essential Oils*, by Kurt Schnaubelt, Ph.D.

THANK YOU

Thank you for reading; I hope this has been helpful for you! If it was beneficial, please consider leaving a review on the book's Amazon listing; that's very helpful to me as an author!

As my gift to you, I've created a printable PDF of the dilution chart in the chapter on carrier oils. Simply visit the following page to find and download it:

titus2homemaker.com/thank-you-for-buying-essentials-of-essential-oils

ABOUT THE AUTHOR

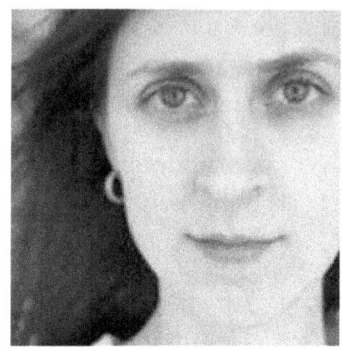

Rachel Ramey is a stay-at-home-mom of four (and a wife!) with a passion for natural and holistic health. She loves research and learning, and she loves to share that knowledge with others.

You can find her online, blogging at Titus2Homemaker, selling essential oils through her Simply Aroma storefront and safe cleaning supplies from Norwex *(at the time of this writing she's an independent consultant for both)*, or pinning, tweeting, and posting to Facebook or Google+

Find Rachel online:
titus2homemaker.com
simplyaroma.com/titus2homemaker
rachelramey.norwex.biz
pinterest.com/titus2homemaker
twitter.com/titus2homemaker
facebook.com/titus2homemaker
plus.google.com/+Titus2Homemaker

REFERENCES

Chemistry of Essential Oils, Dr. David Stewart, Ph.D.
Encyclopedia of Aromatherapy, The, by Chrissie Wildwood
Essential Oils Desk Reference, The, by Connie and Alan Higley
Healing Intelligence of Essential Oils, The, by Kurt Schnaubelt, Ph.D.
Healing Oils of the Bible, Dr. David Stewart, Ph.D.

...and other miscellaneous research done for my own studies over time, which I am no longer able to pinpoint.

www.ingramcontent.com/pod-product-compliance
Lightning Source LLC
Chambersburg PA
CBHW070242290526
45789CB00004B/1725